# Green n' Gluten-Free

On the Go and Snacks Cookbook

## Introduction

Are you free of gluten and looking to get more in touch with the "natural" side of eating? In this recipe book you will find many Gluten-Free No Cook recipes that will help you reach your health improvement goals.

Hunger is the worst enemy of the gluten free diet. It is what compels us to make bad choices sometimes. That's where these No Cook Gluten-Free recipes will really come to the rescue. With a little planning, most of these recipes can be prepared in a jiffy. If you're not out and about, but just looking for a light meal or something to hold you over until the main meal, the items in this book are terrific! Whether you're looking for something salty, spicy, or sweet, we've got you covered!

# Table of Contents

Mango Snacks

Pineapple Chews

Banana Crisps

Sweet Apple Chips

Spicy Kale Crisps

Savory Sweet Potato Chips

Cheesy Popcorn

# Lemon Energy Bars

Prep Time: 25 minutes

Servings: 6

## INGREDIENTS

1 cup raw cashews

2 lemons

1/2 cup dried pineapple

1/2 cup flaked or shredded coconut

1/4 cup dried apricots

1/4 teaspoon ground ginger

1/4 teaspoon vanilla

Pinch Celtic sea salt

1/3 cup warm water

## INSTRUCTIONS

1. Zest *then* juice lemons into small mixing bowl. Reserve half of juice and zest.
2. Soak dried pineapple and apricots in warm water and juice and zest of 1 lemon for 5 - 10 minutes.
3. Line loaf pan with parchment paper.
4. Add cashews to food processor or high-speed blender. Drain fruit and add to processor with coconut, salt, spices, and lemon juice and zest. Process for about 1 minute, until fruit and nuts break down and mixture sticks together when pressed.
5. Transfer mixture to prepared loaf pan and press firmly into bottom with hands or spatula.

6. Place in refrigerator and chill for 10 minutes. Remove and cut into 6 bars.
7. Serve immediately. Or store refrigerated in airtight container up to 2 weeks.

# Ginger Crisps

Prep Time: 5 minutes

Dehydrating Time: 4 - 8 hours

Servings: 12

## INGREDIENTS

2 cups raw almond flour

1 1/2 cups dried pitted dates

4 inch piece fresh ginger

2 tablespoons raw coconut oil (or raw cacao or coconut butter)

2 tablespoons raw honey

2 teaspoons ground ginger

1 teaspoons ground cinnamon

1/2 teaspoon ground black pepper (or ground white pepper)

1/2 teaspoon vanilla

1/4 teaspoon Celtic sea salt

## INSTRUCTIONS

1. Peel and grate ginger. Add to food processor or high-speed blender with almond flour, dates, oil or butter, honey, salt and spices . Process until mixture is well ground and comes together, about 2 minutes.
2. Line dehydrator trays with dehydrator or parchment sheets.
3. Form mixture into 12 - 24 balls and place on lined dehydrator trays. Press to flatten.
4. Place in dehydrator and dehydrate at 115 degrees F for 4 - 8 hours, until desired crispiness is reached.

5. Remove from dehydrator and transfer to serving dish. Serve immediately. Or store in airtight container.

# Crisp Cocoa Wafers

Prep Time: 10 minutes*

Dehydrating Time: 8 - 16 hours

Servings: 12

INGREDIENTS

1/2 cup almonds

3/4 cups cashews

1/3 cup dates

1/4 cup raw cocoa powder

1 tablespoon raw oil (coconut, walnut, almond, sesame, etc.)

1 teaspoon vanilla

1/4 teaspoon Celtic sea salt

Water

INSTRUCTIONS

1. *Soak almonds in enough water to cover for at least 6 hours, or overnight in refrigerator. Drain and rinse. Soak cashews and dates in enough water to cover for at least 1 hour. Drain.
2. Add soaked almonds and cashews to food processor or high-speed blender. Process until finely ground, about 1 - 2 minutes.
3. Add dates, cocoa, oil, vanilla and salt to processor. Process until mixture is well combined and sticks together, about 1 - 2 minutes.
4. Line dehydrator trays with dehydrator or parchment sheets.
5. Form mixture into 12 balls and place on dehydrator or parchment sheets. Press to flatten.

6. Place in dehydrator and dehydrate at 115 degrees F for about 8 - 16 hours, depending on desired crispiness.

7. Remove from dehydrator and transfer to serving dish. Serve immediately. Or store in airtight container.

# Good Morning Trail Mix

Prep Time: 5 minutes

Servings: 4

INGREDIENTS

1/2 cup raw almonds

1/2 cup raw pumpkin seeds

1/2 cup cashews

1/4 cup golden raisins

1/4 cup dried blueberries

1/4 cup dried strawberries

INSTRUCTIONS

1. Roughly chop dried strawberries. Add to medium mixing bowl with fruit and nuts. Mix to combine.
2. Transfer to serving dish and serve immediately. Or store in airtight container.

# Preserved Beef Jerky

Prep Time: 10 minutes*

Dehydrating Time: 4 - 8 hours

Servings: 4

INGREDIENTS

4 oz grass-fed beef

2 tablespoons coconut aminos (or liquid aminos or tamari)

2 tablespoons lemon juice (or raw apple cider vinegar)

1 tablespoons Celtic sea salt

1/2 teaspoon ground ginger

1/2 teaspoon garlic powder

1/2 teaspoon onion powder

1/2 teaspoon smoked paprika

1/2 teaspoon cayenne pepper

INSTRUCTIONS

1. Prepare two parchment sheets. Lay one on cutting board.
2. Cut slice beef into 1/4 inch strips and lay in single layer on parchment. Pound with tenderizing side of kitchen mallet. Cover beef with second parchment sheet, then pound with flat side of tenderizing mallet to 1/8 inch thickness.
3. *Place beef strips in medium mixing bowl or shallow dish. Add coconut aminos, lemon juice, salt and spices. Mix well to coat. Cover and place in refrigerator for 8 hours, or overnight.

4.  Remove beef from refrigerator and lay in single layer on dehydrator trays. Place in dehydrator and dehydrate at 120 degrees F for 4 - 8 hours.

5.  After 4 hours dehydrating time, remove trays from dehydrator and test beef by bending. If it cracks, remove and serve immediately. Or store in airtight container.

6.  If still flexible, place back in dehydrator and continue dehydrating up to 4 hours, or until desired texture is achieved.

# Fruit and Nut Apricot Pockets

Prep Time: 10 minutes

Servings: 4

## INGREDIENTS

1 cup dried apricots

1/4 cup raw cashews

2 - 3 tablespoons dried cranberries

2 - 3 tablespoons dried blueberries

## INSTRUCTIONS

1. Roughly chop cashews and add too small mixing bowl with cranberries and blueberries. Mix to combine.

2. Open apricots slightly to reveal pocket. Take pinch of mixed nuts and fruit and stuff apricots. Leave a little room to pinch apricot closed.

3. Transfer to serving dish and serve immediately. Or store in airtight container.

# Sweet Treat Blondie Bars

Prep Time: 35 minutes

Servings: 6

## INGREDIENTS

1 cup dried pitted dates

1 cup flaked or shredded coconut

3/4 cup golden flax seed

1/2 cup raw sunflower seeds (or raw pine nuts)

1/4 cup cacao butter (or coconut butter)

1/4 teaspoon Celtic sea salt

1 teaspoon vanilla

1/4cup cacao nibs (or raw chocolate chunks) (optional)

## INSTRUCTIONS

1. Line baking dish with parchment paper. Allow cacao butter or coconut butter to soften.
2. Add flax to food processor or high-speed blender and process until finely ground, about 2 minutes. Add sunflower seeds and cacao butter. Process until fairly smooth, about 2 minutes.
3. Add dates, coconut, vanilla and salt. Process until mixture comes together, about 1 minute.
4. Transfer to medium mixing bowl and stir in cacao nibs or raw chocolate chunks (optional).
5. Transfer mixture to lined dish and press into bottom with hands or spatula. Place in freezer at least 25 minutes.

6. Remove from freezer. Slice and serve chilled. Or allow to warm slightly and serve.

# Summer Sweet Bread

Prep Time: 10 minutes

Dehydrating Time: 6 - 8 hours

Servings: 8


INGREDIENTS

1 apple

1 lemon

1 orange

1 cup dried pitted dates

1/2 cup dried apricots

1/3 cup ground flax seed

1/2 cup raw pecans

1/2 cup raw walnuts

1 teaspoon ground cinnamon

1 teaspoon ground ginger

1/4 teaspoon Celtic sea salt


INSTRUCTIONS

1. Add pecans, walnuts and flax to food processor or high-speed blender. Process until finely ground, about 1 minute.
2. Peel and roughly chop apple around core. Zest *then* juice orange and lemon. Add to food processor or high-speed blender with dates, apricots, cinnamon, ginger and salt. Process until mixture is well ground and sticks together, about 2 minutes.
3. Line dehydrator tray with dehydrator or parchment sheet.

4. Form mixture into 2 loaves and place on lined dehydrator tray. Place in dehydrator and dehydrate at 115 degrees F for 2 hours. Reduce to 110 degrees F and continue to dehydrate for another 4 - 6 hours.

5. Remove from dehydrator and slice. Transfer to serving dish and serve immediately. Or store in airtight container.

# Coconut Lemon Biscuits

Prep Time: 5 minutes

Dehydrating Time: 8 - 12 hours

Servings: 12

## INGREDIENTS

1 cup cashews

1 cup flaked or shredded coconut

1 lemon

1 tablespoon raw honey

## INSTRUCTIONS

1. Add cashews to food processor or high-speed blender and process until finely ground, about 1 minute.

2. Zest *then* juice lemon. Add to processor with coconut and honey. Process until mixture is well combined and sticks together, about 1 - 2 minutes.

3. Line dehydrator trays with dehydrator or parchment sheets.

4. Form mixture into 12 - 24 balls and place on dehydrator or parchment sheets. Press to flatten.

5. Place in dehydrator and dehydrate on 115 degrees F for about 8 - 12 hours, until desired crispiness is reached.

6. Remove from dehydrator and transfer to serving dish. Serve immediately. Or store in airtight container.

# Spicy Sesame Crackers

Prep Time: 10 minutes

Dehydrating Time: 12 - 20 hours

Servings: 4

INGREDIENTS

2 cups ground flax seed

2/3 cup whole flax seed

1 1/3 cups raw sunflower seeds

1/2 cup raw black sesame seeds (or white sesame seeds)

1 orange

1 teaspoon ground cinnamon

1 teaspoon ground ginger

1 teaspoon ground black pepper (or ground white pepper)

1 teaspoon Celtic sea salt

2 2/3 cups water

INSTRUCTIONS

1. Place parchment paper or dehydrator sheets on dehydrator trays.

2. Zest *then* juice orange and add to large mixing bowl with water, seeds, salt and spices. Mix until well combined.

3. Spread batter on lined dehydrator trays. Place trays in dehydrator and set to 120 degrees F for 1 hour. Reduce temperature to 105 degrees F for 12 - 20.

4. After 4 hours, remove trays from dehydrator and use knife to score crackers in preferred shape and size. Place back in dehydrator and continue dehydrating.

5.  Remove trays from dehydrator. Peel crackers from sheets and break apart along score lines. Place crackers directly on dehydrator tray and continue dehydrating another 6 - 12 hours, depending on desired crispness.

6.  Remove crackers from dehydrator and serve immediately. Or store in an airtight container.

# Cheesy Kale Crisps

Prep Time: 10 minutes

Cook Time: 12 - 24 hours

Servings: 8

## INGREDIENTS

2 cups raw almonds

1 kale head (about 3 cups chopped)

1 cup raw coconut flour

1 cup golden flax seed

1 cup water

3/4 cup nutritional yeast

1/2 teaspoon ground black pepper

1 teaspoon smoked paprika

1 teaspoon Celtic sea salt

## INSTRUCTIONS

1. Place parchment paper or dehydrator sheets on dehydrator trays.
2. Add flax to food processor or high-speed blender and process until finely ground, about 2 minutes. Transfer to small mixing bowl with water. Mix to combine and set aside.
3. Add almonds to food processor or high-speed blender and process until finely ground, about 2 minutes. Transfer to medium mixing bowl.
4. Wash and spin dry kale. Add to processor and pulse to finely chop, about 1 minute. Add to mixing bowl with nutritional yeast, salt and spices. Add soaked flax and mix until dough forms.

5. Transfer dough to lined dehydrator trays and press into 1/4 inch thick rectangle with hands or rolling pin. Score with knife or pizza cutter into desired shapes.

6. Place tray in dehydrator and dehydrate at 120 degrees F for 2 hours. Reduce temperature to 115 degrees F and continue to dehydrate for 8 - 12 hours.

7. After 6 hours, remove trays from dehydrator and flip crackers. Place back in dehydrator and continue dehydrating .

8. Remove crackers from dehydrator and serve immediately. Or store in airtight container.

# Spicy Jalapeño Poppers

Prep Time: 20 minutes*

Dehydrating Time: 8 - 24 hours

Servings: 2

INGREDIENTS

6 fresh jalapeño peppers

*Filling*

1 cup raw sunflower seeds

1/2 cup water

1/4 cup nutritional yeast

1 lemon

1 teaspoon onion powder

1 teaspoon Celtic sea salt

Water

*Breading*

1/2 cup raw almonds

1/2 teaspoon Celtic sea salt

1/2 teaspoon ground white pepper (or ground black pepper)

1/2 teaspoon garlic powder (optional)

1/2 teaspoon onion powder (optional)

INSTRUCTIONS

1.  *Soak sunflower seeds in enough water to cover for 2 hours. Drain and rinse.

2. Cut jalapeños in half lengthwise and remove stems, seeds and veins. Place peppers on dehydrator tray.

3. For *Filling*, juice lemon and add to food processor or high-speed blender with soaked sunflower seeds, water, nutritional yeast, salt, pepper and spices. Process until thick, smooth paste forms, about 2 minutes.

4. Fill piping bag with mixture and pipe into jalapeño halves. Or use teaspoon to scoop filling into jalapeño halves.

5. For *Breading*, add raw almonds to clean food processor orhigh-speed blender with salt and spices. Process until well ground but some texture remains, about 30 seconds.

6. Dip stuffed peppers filling-side down into bread and coat generously.

7. Place stuffed and coated peppers on dehydrator tray filling-side up. Place in dehydrator and dehydrate at 110 degrees F  for 8 - 24 hours, depending on desired texture.

8. Remove peppers from dehydrator and scrve immediately.

# Savory Pepperdew Poppers

Prep Time: 15 minutes

Dehydrating Time: 4 - 8 hours

Servings: 2


INGREDIENTS

6 - 8 pepperdew peppers


*Pine Nut Filling*

1/4 cup raw tahini (or 6 tablespoons raw sesame seeds)

1/4 cup + 2 tablespoons raw pine nuts

1 tablespoon raw oil  (coconut, walnut, almond, sesame, etc.)

1 tablespoon nutritional yeast

Juice of 1/2 lemon

1/2 teaspoon ground white pepper (or ground black pepper)

1/2 teaspoon Celtic sea salt


INSTRUCTIONS

1. Cut tops off of peppers and scoop out seeds. Set aside.
2. Add tahini or sesame seeds, 1/4 cup pine nuts, oil,  nutritional yeast, lemon juice, salt and pepper to food processor or high-speed blender. Process until smooth and creamy, up to 5 minutes.
1. Scoop *Pine Nut Filling* into peppers and top with reserved pine nuts. Press pine nuts into stuffing to seal opening.
2. Place filled peppers in dehydrator and dehydrate at 110 degrees F for 4 - 8 hours, until dried but still moist.

3. Remove peppers from dehydrator and transfer to serving dish. Serve immediately. Or store in airtight container.

# Fruity Granola Bars

Prep Time: 30 minutes

Servings: 8

## INGREDIENTS

1 cup raw cashews (or 3/4 cup raw cashew butter)

2 tablespoons flax seed (or chia seed)

1/2 cup dried pitted dates

1/2 cup shredded or flaked coconut

1/3 cup raw pumpkin seeds

1/3 cup raw walnuts

1/3 cup raw almonds

1/4 cup dried cherries

1/4 cup dried blueberries

1/4cup dried raspberries

1/2 teaspoon ground ginger (optional)

1/2 teaspoon vanilla

1 teaspoon Celtic sea salt

## INSTRUCTIONS

1. Line loaf pan with parchment paper.
2. Add flax or chia to food processor or high-speed blender and process until finely ground, about 1 - 2 minutes.
3. Add cashews (if using)and process until thick, smooth paste forms, up to 5 minutes.
4. Add dates and process until thick, fairly smooth mixture forms about 1 - 2 minutes. Transfer to medium mixing bowl.

5. Add coconut, pumpkin seeds, walnuts, almonds, vanilla, salt, dried fruit and ginger (optional). Add prepared cashew butter (if using). Stir to combine with large wooden spoon.

6. Transfer mixture to parchment lined pan and firmly press into bottom with hands or spatula. Place in refrigerator for 20 minutes.

7. Remove from refrigerator and cut into bars. Serve chilled. Or allow to warm to room temperature and serve.

# Banana Berry Fruit Rolls

Prep Time: 5 minutes

Dehydrating Time: 6 hours

Servings: 6

## INGREDIENTS

1 ripe banana

2 cups fresh strawberries (chopped)

2 tablespoons ground chia or flax seed (optional)

Water (optional)

## INSTRUCTIONS

1. Remove stems from fresh strawberries and roughly chop. Peel and chop banana. Add to food processor or high-speed blender and process until smooth, about 1 minute.

2. Add ground chia or flax to processor and process with enough water to reach desired consistency. Mixture should be spreadable but not runny.

3. Line dehydrator tray with dehydrator or parchment sheet.

4. Spread mixture on sheet 1/4 inch thick in large rectangle with spatula. Place in dehydrator and dehydrate at 115 degrees F for 4 hours.

5. Remove from dehydrator and use offset spatula to gently peel leather from sheet and flip over. Place back in dehydrator directly on tray and continue to dehydrate for 2 hours.

6. Remove from dehydrator and cut into strips. Or roll up and cut into logs. Transfer to serving dish and serve immediately.

# Crispy Carrot Chips

Prep Time: 5 minutes

Dehydrating Time: 18 - 24 hours

Servings: 4

INGREDIENTS

2 large carrots

1 tablespoon raw oil (coconut, walnut, almond, sesame, etc.) (optional)

1/2 teaspoon Celtic sea salt (optional)

INSTRUCTIONS

1. Carefully cut carrot into 1/16 - 1/8 inch thick slices with sharp knife, mandolin or food processor with slicing attachment.
2. Add sliced carrot to medium mixing bowl with oil and salt and toss to coat (optional).
3. Add single layer of sliced carrots to dehydrator tray and place in dehydrator. Dehydrate at 115 degrees F for 12 hours.
4. Remove dehydrator trays and turn over carrot slices. Place trays back in dehydrator and continue dehydrating for 6 - 12 hours, depending on desired crispiness.
5. Remove carrots from dehydrator and transfer to serving dish. Serve immediately. Or store in airtight container.

# Acorn Squash Crisps

Prep Time: 5 minutes

Dehydrating Time: 18 - 24 hours

Servings: 4

## INGREDIENTS

1 acorn squash

1 tablespoon raw oil (coconut, walnut, almond, sesame, etc.) (optional)

1/4 teaspoon smoked paprika

1/4 teaspoon ground white pepper (or ground black pepper)

1/4 teaspoon Italian seasoning blend (optional)

1/2 teaspoon Celtic sea salt

## INSTRUCTIONS

1. Carefully cut acorn squash into 1/16 - 1/8 inch thick slices with sharp knife, mandolin or food processor with slicing attachment.
2. Add sliced squash to medium mixing bowl with oil, salt and spices. Toss to coat.
3. Add single layer of sliced squash to dehydrator tray and place in dehydrator. Dehydrate at 115 degrees F for 12 hours.
4. Remove dehydrator trays and turn over squash slices. Place trays back in dehydrator and continue dehydrating for 6 - 12 hours, depending on desired crispiness.
5. Remove squash from dehydrator and transfer to serving dish. Serve immediately. Or store in airtight container.

# Confetti Beet Chips

Prep Time: 15 minutes

Dehydrating Time: 18 - 24 hours

Servings: 4


INGREDIENTS

2 red beets

2 golden beets (or 2 red beets)

1/4 cup water

1/4 cup raw apple cider vinegar

1 tablespoon raw oil (coconut, walnut, almond, sesame, etc.)

1 teaspoon Celtic seat salt

1/2 teaspoon ground black pepper


INSTRUCTIONS

1. Wash and scrub beets. Carefully cut into 1/16 - 1/8 inch thick slices with sharp knife, mandolin or food processor with slicing attachment.
2. Add sliced beets to medium mixing bowl with water, vinegar and oil. Toss to coat. Set aside 10 minutes.
3. Drain beets, then sprinkle on salt and pepper. Toss to coat.
4. Add single layer of beets to dehydrator tray and place in dehydrator. Dehydrate at 115 degrees F for 12 hours.
5. Remove dehydrator trays and turn over beet slices. Place trays back in dehydrator and continue dehydrating for 12 hours, depending on desired crispiness.

6. Remove beets from dehydrator and transfer to serving dish. Serve immediately. Or store in airtight container.

# Mango Snacks

Prep Time: 10 minutes

Dehydrating Time: 24 hours

Servings: 4


INGREDIENTS

2 ripe mangos


INSTRUCTIONS

1. Cut mango around pit, and cut into 1/4 inch thick slices. Then remove peel. Or slice then peel.
2. Add single layer of sliced mango to dehydrator trays. Place in dehydrator and dehydrate at 115 degrees F for 24 hours, or until dried but not crisp.
3. Remove mango from dehydrator and transfer to serving dish. Serve immediately. Or store in airtight container.

# Pineapple Chews

Prep Time: 10 minutes

Dehydrating Time: 12 - 16 hours

Servings: 4

INGREDIENTS

1 ripe pineapple

INSTRUCTIONS

1. Peel pineapple and cut around core into 1/4 - 1/3 inch thick slices.
2. Add single layer of sliced pineapple to dehydrator trays. Place in dehydrator and dehydrate at 115 degrees F for 12 - 16 hours, or until dried but not crisp.
3. Remove pineapple from dehydrator and transfer to serving dish. Serve immediately. Or store in airtight container.

# Banana Crisps

Prep Time: 5 minutes

Dehydrating Time: 12 - 16 hours

Servings: 4

INGREDIENTS

4 ripe or overripe bananas

INSTRUCTIONS

1. Peel bananas and cut into 1/4 - 1/3 inch thick slices lengthwise or crosswise.
2. Line dehydrator trays with dehydrator or parchment sheet. Add single layer of sliced banana to lined dehydrator trays .
3. Place bananas in dehydrator and dehydrate on 115 degrees F for 12 - 16 hours, depending on desired crispiness.
4. Remove bananas from dehydrator and transfer to serving dish. Serve immediately. Or store in airtight container.

# Sweet Apple Chips

Prep Time: 5 minutes

Dehydrating Time: 10 - 14 hours

Servings: 4

INGREDIENTS

4 sweet apples

1 teaspoon ground cinnamon (optional)

INSTRUCTIONS

1. Carefully cut apple around core into 1/16 - 1/8 inch thick slices with sharp knife, mandolin or food processor with slicing attachment.

2. Add single layer of sliced apple to dehydrator tray . Sprinkle with cinnamon (optional). Place in dehydrator and dehydrate at 105 degrees F for 10 - 14 hours, depending on desired crispiness.

3. Remove apples from dehydrator and transfer to serving dish. Serve immediately. Or store in airtight container.

# Spicy Kale Crisps

Prep Time: 10 minutes

Dehydrating Time: 4 - 6 hours

Servings: 4

## INGREDIENTS

2 kale heads (or 1.5 - 2 lbs kale leaves)

3 tablespoons raw oil (coconut, walnut, almond, sesame, etc.)

1 tablespoon coconut aminos (or tamari, apple cider vinegar or lemon juice)

1/2 teaspoon smoked paprika

1 teaspoon cayenne pepper

1 teaspoon ground black pepper

1 teaspoon Celtic sea salt

## INSTRUCTIONS

1. Wash and spin dry kale. Remove tough spine and chop or tear into pieces.
2. Add kale pieces to large mixing bowl with oil, vinegar salt and spices. Toss to coat.
3. Add single layer of coated kale to dehydrator tray and place in dehydrator. Dehydrate at 115 degrees F for 4 - 6 hours, depending on desired crispiness.
4. Remove kale from dehydrator and transfer to serving dish. Serve immediately. Or store in airtight container.

# Savory Sweet Potato Chips

Prep Time: 5 minutes

Dehydrating Time: 24 hours

Servings: 4

## INGREDIENTS

1 large sweet potato

2 tablespoons raw oil (coconut, walnut, almond, sesame, etc.)

1 teaspoon Celtic sea salt

1/2 teaspoon ground black pepper (optional)

## INSTRUCTIONS

1. Carefully cut sweet potato into 1/16 - 1/8 inch thick slices with sharp knife, mandolin or food processor with slicing attachment.
2. Add sliced sweet potato to medium mixing bowl with oil, salt and pepper. Toss to coat.
3. Add single layer of coated sweet potatoes to dehydrator tray and place in dehydrator. Dehydrate at 115 degrees F for 12 hours.
4. Remove dehydrator trays and turn over sweet potato slices. Place trays back in dehydrator and continue dehydrating for about 12 hours, depending on desired crispiness.
5. Remove sweet potatoes from dehydrator and transfer to serving dish. Serve immediately. Or store in airtight container.

# Cheesy

## Popcorn Prep Time: 5 minutes

Dehydrating Time: 12 - 24
hours Servings: 2

### INGREDIENTS

2 cups cauliflower florets (roughly chopped)

1 teaspoon raw oil (coconut, walnuts, almond, sesame, etc.)

1 teaspoon coconut aminos (or tamari, apple cider vinegar or lemon
juice)

3 tablespoons nutritional yeast

1 teaspoon Celtic sea salt

### INSTRUCTIONS

1. Cut larger cauliflower florets into smaller pieces. Add to medium mixing bowl or container with well-fitting lid.
2. Evenly sprinkle on oil, coconut aminos, nutritional yeast and salt.
3. Secure lid on bowl or container and shake well until cauliflower is

   evenly coated.
4. Line dehydrator trays with dehydrator or parchment sheets.
5. Add single layer of coated cauliflower to lined dehydrator trays and place in dehydrator. Dehydrate at 115 degrees F for 12 - 24 hours, until desired crispiness is reached.  Turn cauliflower over half way through dehydrating.
6. Remove from dehydrator and transfer to serving dish. Serve immediately.

# Snacks Cookbook

# Table of Contents

Chocolate Chia Pudding

Coconut Rice Pudding

Nori with Almond Cheese

Quick Asian Slaw

Awesome Strawberry Salsa

Supreme Mango Salsa

Hot Apricot Pineapple Salsa

Fresh Zesty Pico de Gallo

Holy Loaded Guacamole

Spicy Stuffed Jalapeños

# Crisp Sesame Crackers

Prep Time: 10 minutes

Dehydrating Time: 12 - 20 hours

Servings: 4

## INGREDIENTS

2 cups ground flax seed

2/3 cup whole flax seed

1 1/3 cups raw sunflower seeds

1/2 cup raw black sesame seeds (or white sesame seeds)
Small bunch fresh parsley

1/4 teaspoon dried basil

1/4 teaspoon onion powder

1/4 teaspoon garlic powder

1 teaspoon Celtic sea salt

2 2/3 cups water

## INSTRUCTIONS

1. Place parchment paper or dehydrator sheets on two dehydrator trays.

2. Finely mince fresh parsley. Add to large mixing bowl with seeds, salt and spices. Mix until well combined.

3. Spread batter on prepared sheets. Place trays in dehydrator and set to 120 degrees F for 1 hour. Reduce temperature to 105 degrees F for remainder of dehydrating time.

2. After 4 hours dehydrating time, remove trays from dehydrator and use knife to score crackers in preferred shape and size. Placeback in dehydrator and continue dehydrating another 4 hours.

3. Remove trays from dehydrator. Peel crackers from sheets and break apart along score lines. Place crackers directly on dehydrator tray and continue dehydrating another 4 - 12 hours, depending on desired crispness.

4. Remove crackers from dehydrator and serve with your favorite raw dips, spreads and salsas. Or store in an airtight container up to 4 weeks.

# Veggie Flax Crackers

Prep Time: 10 minutes

Cook Time: 12 - 24 hours

Servings: 4

## INGREDIENTS

1 medium tomato

1 medium onion

2 medium zucchini

1 cup ground flax seed

2 tablespoons coconut aminos (or raw apple cider vinegar)

1/2 teaspoon ground black pepper

1 teaspoon Celtic sea salt

## INSTRUCTIONS

1. Place parchment paper or dehydrator sheets on two dehydrator trays.

2. Peel onion and chop. Chop zucchini and tomato. Add to food processor or high-speed blender with flax meal, coconut aminos or vinegar, salt and pepper. Process until well ground, about 2 minutes.

3. Spread batter on prepared sheets. Place trays in dehydrator and set to 120 degrees F for 1 hour. Reduce temperature to 105 degrees F for remainder of dehydrating time.

4. After 4 hours dehydrating time, remove trays from dehydrator and use knife to score crackers in preferred shape and size. Place back in dehydrator and continue dehydrating another 4 hours.

6.  Remove trays from dehydrator. Peel crackers from sheets and break apart along score lines. Place crackers directly on dehydrator tray and continue dehydrating another 4 - 12 hours, depending on desired crispness.

7.  Remove crackers from dehydrator and serve with your favorite raw dips, spreads and salsas. Or store in an airtight container up to 4 weeks.

# Avocado Cashew Hummus with Cucumber

Prep Time: 5 minutes*

Servings: 4


INGREDIENTS 1

cup raw cashews

1 avocado

Juice of 1/2 lemon

2 garlic cloves

1 teaspoon ground white pepper (or 1/2 teaspoon ground black pepper) Small bunch fresh cilantro

1/2 teaspoon Celtic sea

salt 1small cucumber

Water


## INSTRUCTIONS

1. *Soak cashews in enough water to cover at least 4 hours, or overnight in refrigerator. Drain and rinse.

2. Peel garlic. Juice lemon. Remove cilantro leaves from stem. Add to food processor or high-speed blender with soaked cashews, salt and pepper.

3. Slice avocado in half. Remove pit and scoop flesh into processor. Process until smooth, about 1 -2 minutes. Add water or raw oil to reach desired consistency, if necessary.

4. Transfer mixture to serving dish.

1. Peel cucumber if desired. Cut diagonally into 1/3 inch slices. Arrange on serving dish.

2. Serve immediately with hummus. Or place in refrigerator for 20 minutes, then serve chilled.

# Sundried Tomato Cashew Hummus with Carrots

Prep Time: 5 minutes*

Servings: 4

## INGREDIENTS

1 1/2 cup raw cashews 1/4
cup sundried tomatoes

1/4 cup raw tahini (or 1/3 cup raw sesame seeds)
1/2 lemon

1 small garlic clove

1 teaspoon ground white pepper (or 1/2 teaspoon ground black pepper)
1/2 teaspoon Celtic sea salt

2 large carrots
Water

## INSTRUCTIONS

1. *Soak cashews in enough water to cover at least 4 hours, or overnight in refrigerator. Drain and rinse.

2. Peel garlic. Juice lemon. Add to food processor or high-speed blender with raw sesame seeds and process until smooth, if using.

3. Or add tahini to processor with soaked cashews, sundried tomatoes, garlic, lemon juice, salt and pepper. Process until smooth, about 1 -2 minutes. Add water or raw oil to reach desired consistency, if necessary.

4. Transfer mixture to serving dish.

5. Peel carrots if desired. Cut into 4 inch long x 1/2 inch thick sticks. Arrange on serving dish.
6. Serve immediately with hummus. Or place in refrigerator for 20 minutes, then serve chilled.

# Cocoa Date Spread

Prep Time: 5 minutes*

Servings: 4

## INGREDIENTS

10 - 12 oz dried pitted dates

2 cups water

3 tablespoons raw cocoa powder

1/2 teaspoon ground cinnamon

1/4 teaspoon ground ginger

Ground black pepper, to taste

## INSTRUCTIONS

1.  *Soak dates in water overnight. Drain and reserve 1/4 cup liquid.

2.  Add soaked dates, cocoa powder, cinnamon, ginger and black pepper to taste to food processor or high-speed blender. Pulse until chunky mixture forms. Add reserved liquid to reach desired consistency, if necessary.

3.  Or add dates to medium mixing bowl with cocoa powder, cinnamon, ginger and black pepper to taste. Mash with large fork or potato masher for about 5 minutes, until chunky mixture forms. Add reserved liquid to reach desired consistency, if necessary.

4.  Transfer to serving dish and serve with fruits, veggies, or raw crackers and breads.

# Cashew Spinach Dip with Bell Pepper

Prep Time: 10 minutes

Servings: 2

## INGREDIENTS

2 - 3 cups spinach leaves

1 1/2 cups raw cashews

3 garlic cloves

1 lemon

1/3 cup water

1/4 teaspoon mustard powder (or mustard seeds)

1/2 teaspoon ground white pepper (or 1/4 teaspoon ground black pepper)

1/2 teaspoon Celtic sea salt

1 red bell pepper

## INSTRUCTIONS

1   Cut bell pepper in half and remove seeds, veins and stems. Slice peppers into 1 - 1 1/2 inch strips. Arrange on serving dish and set aside.

2   Juice lemon. Peel garlic. Add to food processor or high-speed blender with cashews and mustard powder or seeds. Process until finely ground, about 2 minutes.

3   Add salt, pepper and water. Process until smooth. Add spinach and pulse until spinach is desired texture.

4   Transfer mixture to serving dish. Serving immediately with bell pepper slices. Or refrigerate 20 minutes and serve chilled.

# Chocolate Hazelnut Spread with Apples

Prep Time: 5 minutes*

Servings: 2

## INGREDIENTS

1 cup raw hazelnuts

1/4 cup raw cocoa powder

1/4 cup raw honey (or dried pitted dates)
2/3 teaspoon vanilla

1/4 teaspoon Celtic sea
salt 2 apples

Raw nut milk (optional)

Water

## INSTRUCTIONS

1. *Soak hazelnuts in enough water to cover overnight in refrigerator. Soak dates in enough water to cover overnight in refrigerator, if using. Drain and rinse.

2. Add soaked hazelnuts to food processor or high-speed blender and process until smooth, up to 10 minutes. Scrape down sides as needed.

3. Add honey or soaked dates, cocoa powder, vanilla and salt. Process until smooth, about 1 minute. Add nut milk to reach desired consistency, if necessary.

4. Transfer mixture to serving dish.

5. Remove core, seeds and stems from apples. Slice into wedges and arrange on serving dish. Serve immediately.

# Cashew Butter Date Snacks

Prep Time: 5 minutes

Servings: 2

## INGREDIENTS

6 whole dried pitted dates
Pinch ground cinnamon

*Raw Cashew Butter*

1 cup raw cashews

1 dried pitted date

1 teaspoon raw oil (coconut, walnut, almond, sesame, etc.)
1/2 teaspoon ground cinnamon

1/4 teaspoon Celtic sea salt

(or 1/2 cup prepared raw cashew butter)

## INSTRUCTIONS

1. For *Cashew Butter*, add cashews, date, cinnamon, salt and oil to food processor or high-speed blender. Process until smooth, up to 5 minutes. Let mixture rest between periods of processing to reach desired consistency, if necessary.
2. Slice dates in half lengthwise. Use small spoon to fill date halves with prepared or *Raw Cashew Butter*. Sprinkle ground cinnamon over filled dates.
3. Arrange on serving dish and serve immediately.

# Very Cherry Energy Bars

Prep Time: 25 minutes

Servings: 6

## INGREDIENTS

1 cup dried cherries

1/4 cup dried pitted dates
1 cup raw almonds

1/4 teaspoon ground cinnamon
1/4 teaspoon vanilla

1/8 teaspoon Celtic sea salt
1/3 cup warm water

1/2 sour orange (or orange or tangerine)

## INSTRUCTIONS

1. Zest and juice orange into small mixing bowl. Add warm water and dried cherries. Toss to coat and set aside 10 minutes.

2. Line loaf pan with parchment paper.

3. Add nuts and dates to food processor or high-speed blender. Drain soaked cherries and add to processor with cinnamon, vanilla and salt. Process for about 1 minute, until mixture is coarsely ground and sticks together when pressed.

4. Scrape mixture into prepared loaf pan and press firmly into bottom with hands or spatula.

5. Place in refrigerator and chill for 10 minutes. Remove and cut into 6 bars.

6. Serve immediately. Or store in refrigerator up to 2 weeks.

# Sweet Coconut Ambrosia Salad

Prep Time: 15 minutes*

Servings: 2


INGREDIENTS

3 mature coconuts

1 1/2 cups water

6 clementines or tangerines (about 1 cup segments)

1 cup fresh pineapple (chopped)

1 cup pecans (chopped)

1 cup fresh cherries (pitted)


INSTRUCTIONS

1. Remove coconut flesh from shells. Add 1 coconut and water to food processor or high-speed blender. Process until well blended and fairly smooth, about 1- 2 minutes.

2. Strain mixture through nut milk bag, cheesecloth or strainer into container. Add coconut milk back to blender with flesh of 2nd coconut. Process again until well blended and thick, about 1 - 2 minutes.

3. Strain mixture through nut milk bag, cheesecloth or strainer into container. Reserve pulp and set aside to dry and dehydrate, then use as coconut flour.

4. *For thicker coconut cream, set aside thickened milk in refrigerator about 20 minutes and allow fat to separate. Remove coconut cream from refrigerator and scoop out risen fat into medium mixing bowl.

5. Or add coconut cream milk to medium mixing bowl. Peel oranges or tangerines and remove segments. Peel pineapple and chop. Cut cherries in half and pit. Chop pecans. Add to coconut cream.

6. Add remaining coconut flesh to clean food processor with shredding attachment and process, or grate with grater. Add coconut to mixture. Stir to combine.

7. Cover mixture and place in refrigerator for 2 hours. Remove and transfer to serving dishes.

8. Serve chilled.

# Sweet Carrot Raisin Salad

Prep Time: 5 minutes

Servings: 2

## INSTRUCTIONS

2 large carrots

2 tablespoons red raisins

2 tablespoons golden raisins

1/4 cup raw slivered almonds (or sliced almonds)

1/2 small orange (or tangerine)

1/4 teaspoon ground cinnamon

## DIRECTIONS

1. Add carrots to food processor with shredding attachment and process, or grate with grater. Add to medium mixing bowl with raisins, almonds and cinnamon.

2. Zest *then* juice orange. Add to carrot mixture and toss to combine.

3. Transfer to serving dishes and serve immediately. Or refrigerate 20 minutes and serve chilled.

# Sweet Coconut Rice with Mango

Prep Time: 10 minutes*

Servings: 2


## INSTRUCTIONS

1 fresh coconut (or 2/3 cup desiccated, shredded or flaked coconut)
1/4 cup raw honey (or 1/4 cup dried pitted dates)

1/4 teaspoon ground ginger (or 1/4 inch piece fresh ginger)
1 mango


## INGREDIENTS

1. *Soak dried coconut and dried pitted dates in enough water to cover overnight in refrigerator, if using. Drain coconut and add to medium mixing bowl. Drain dates and reserve 2 tablespoons soaking liquid.

2. Or remove fresh coconut flesh from shell and add to food processor with shredding attachment and process, or grate with grater. Add to medium mixing bowl.

3. Add soaked dates and soaking liquid to clean food processor or high-speed and process until smooth, if using.

4. Peel fresh ginger and mince or finely grate, if using. Add raw honey or date purée to shredded coconut with ground or fresh ginger. Mix to combine. Transfer to serving dishes.

5. Slice mango in half around pit. Remove peel and diceor thinly slice flesh. Add over sweet shredded coconut.

6. Serve immediately. Or refrigerate 20 minutes and serve chilled.

# Sweet Almond Crunch Cookies

Prep Time: 20 minutes

Servings: 12

## INGREDIENTS

3/4 cup raw almond butter (or 1 cup raw almonds)

2 - 4 tablespoons raw honey (or 1/4 cup dried pitted dates)

1 tablespoon ground chia seed or flax meal (or whole seeds)

1 teaspoon cinnamon

1/2 teaspoon Celtic sea salt

1/4 cup raw almonds

## INSTRUCTIONS

1. Line baking dish with parchment paper.
2. Add 1/4 cup raw almonds to food processor or high-speed blender and process until finely chopped. Set aside.
3. Add whole chia or flax seeds to high-speed blender or spice grinder and grind to fine powder, if using.
4. Add chia or flax meal to food processor or high-speed blender with remaining almonds or almond butter, honey or dates, cinnamon and salt. Process until smooth, thick paste forms, up to 5 minutes. Let mixture rest between periods of processing to reach desired consistency, if necessary.
5. Spread mixture in parchment lined dish. Place in refrigerator or freezer for 10 minutes.
6. Remove dish and scoop with tablespoon or melon baller. Roll into balls with hands.

7. Place chopped almonds in shallow dish and roll balls in almonds to coat.

8. Transfer coated almond cookies to serving dish. Serve immediately. Or refrigerate 20 minutes and serve chilled.

# Chewy Ginger Cookies

Prep Time: 20 minutes*

Servings: 12


INGREDIENTS

1/2 cup raw cashews (frozen)

1 1/2 cups dried pitted dates (1 cup chopped)

2 inch piece fresh ginger

1 teaspoon ground ginger

1/4 teaspoon ground cinnamon

1/2 cup unsweetened flaked or shredded coconut


INSTRUCTIONS

1. * Place cashews in freezer for a few hours to overnight.

2. Add frozen nuts to food processor or high-speed blender. Pulse until coarsely ground.

3. Peel and finely grate fresh ginger. Add to processor with dates, ground ginger and cinnamon. Process until mixture is well broken down and sticks together.

4. Form mixture into 12 balls. Add coconut flakes to shallow dish. Roll ballain coconut until well coated, then gently press to flatten slightly.

5. Arrange on serving dish and cover. Place in freezer for at least 10 minutes, until set up and firm.

6. Remove from freezer and serve chilled. Or store in freezer or refrigerator.

# Chocolate Dusted Almonds

Prep Time: 20 minutes*

Servings: 2

## INGREDIENTS

1 cup raw almonds

1 tablespoon raw cocoa powder

1 tablespoon raw honey

1/8 teaspoon ground
cinnamon 1/8 teaspoon vanilla

## INSTRUCTIONS

1. Add almonds and honey to small mixing bowl and toss to combine.
2. Add cocoa, cinnamon and vanilla and toss to evenly coat.
3. Transfer to serving dish and serve immediately.

# Chocolate Chia Pudding

Prep Time: 15 minutes

Servings: 2

## INGREDIENTS

1 cup nutmilk (or 2 mature coconuts + 1 1/2 cups water) 2

- 4 tablespoons raw honey (or dried pitted dates)

2 - 4 tablespoons whole chia seeds

2 - 3 tablespoons cocoa powder

1/2 teaspoon vanilla

## INSTRUCTIONS

1. Remove coconut flesh from shells. Add 1 coconut and water to food processor or high-speed blender. Process until well blended and fairly smooth, about 1- 2 minutes.

2. Strain mixture through nut milk bag, cheesecloth or strainer into container. Add coconut milk back to blender with remaining coconut flesh. Process again until well blended and fairly smooth, about 1 minute.

3. Strain mixture through nut milk bag, cheesecloth or strainer into container. Reserve pulp and set aside to dry and dehydrate, then use as coconut flour.

4. Add nut milk to high-speed blender with dates and process until smooth, if using.

5. Or add nut milk to small mixing bowl with honey or stevia, cocoa powder, vanilla and chia seeds. Whisk to combine. Set aside to thicken, about 1 minute.

6. Pour mixture into serving dishes and serve immediately. Or refrigerate 20 minutes and serve chilled.

# Coconut Rice Pudding

Prep Time: 20 minutes

Servings: 4

## INGREDIENTS

3 fresh coconuts (or 2 cups unsweetened flaked or shredded coconut)
1 cup water

1/4 - 1/2 cup raw honey (or dried pitted dates)
1 teaspoon vanilla

Water

## INSTRUCTIONS

1. *Soak 1 1/2 cups flaked coconut and dates in enough water to cover in refrigerator overnight. Then drain, if using.

2. Or remove fresh coconut flesh from shells.

3. Add flesh of 1 fresh coconut or 3/4 cup soaked coconut, and water to high-speed blender. Process until well blended and fairly smooth, about 1- 2 minutes.

4. Strain mixture through nut milk bag, cheesecloth or strainer into container. Add coconut milk back to blender with flesh of 1 fresh coconut or remaining soaked coconut. Process again until well blended and fairly smooth, about 1 minute.

5. Strain mixture through nut milk bag, cheesecloth or strainer into container. Reserve pulp and set aside to dry and dehydrate, then use as coconut flour.

6. Add coconut cream, soaked dates and vanilla to food processor or high-speed blender. Process until smooth, about 1 minute.

7. Or add coconut cream to medium mixing bowl with raw honey and vanilla.

8. Add remaining fresh coconut flesh to food processer with shredding attachment and process, or shred with grater.

9. Add shredded fresh coconut or flaked coconut to coconut cream mixture and whisk until well combined.

10. Pour into serving dishes and serve immediately. Or refrigerate for 20 minutes and serve chilled.

# Nori with Almond Cheese

Prep Time: 15 minutes*

Servings: 2

## INGREDIENTS

4 - 6 sheets dried nori (seaweed paper)

*Almond cheese*

1 cup raw almonds

2 tablespoons raw oil (coconut, walnut, almond, sesame, etc.)

2 tablespoons lemon juice (or raw apple cider vinegar)

1 garlic clove

1/4 teaspoon paprika

1/4 teaspoon ground white pepper (or ground black pepper)

1/2 teaspoon Celtic sea salt

Water

## INSTRUCTIONS

1. *For *Almond Cheese*, soak almonds in enough water to cover overnight. Drain and rinse. Pop off skins and discard.

2. Peel garlic and add to food processor or high-speed blender with soaked almonds, oil, lemon juice and/or vinegar, salt and spices. Process until smooth, about 2 minutes. Add water to reach desired consistency, if necessary.

3. Transfer mixture to small serving dish. Cut nori into small sheets and arrange on serving dish.

4. Serve immediately. Or refrigerate for 20 minutes and serve chilled.

# Quick Asian Slaw

Prep Time: 15 minutes*

Servings: 4

## INGREDIENTS

1/2 head red cabbage (2 cups shredded)

2 broccoli stalks (2 cups shredded)

1/4 cup dried cranberries

1/4 cup raw sliced or slivered almonds

2 tablespoons raw sunflower seeds

2 green onions (scallions)

1.carrot

4.lemon

1/2 orange

5.tablespoons raw honey

2 tablespoons raw sesame oil (or coconut, walnut, almond oil, etc.)

2 tablespoons apple cider vinegar

1/2 teaspoon ground ginger

1 teaspoon ground white pepper (or black pepper)

1 teaspoon Celtic sea salt

## INSTRUCTIONS

1. Add broccoli and carrot to food processor with shredding attachment, or grate with grater. Slice green onions. Shred cabbage. Add to large mixing bowl.

2. Add cranberries, almonds, sunflower seeds, honey, oil, vinegar, ginger, salt, pepper and squeeze of lemon and orange. Mix until well combined.
3. *Transfer mixture and for 90 minutes. Serve chilled.

# Awesome Strawberry Salsa

Prep Time: 5 minutes*

Servings: 4


## INGREDIENTS

2 cups fresh strawberries

1/2 small white onion

1/4 red bell pepper

Medium bunch fresh mint

1/2 lime

1/2 orange

1/2 teaspoon ground black pepper


## INSTRUCTIONS

1   Remove strawberry stems and leaves, then finely dice. Add to medium mixing bowl.

2   Peel onion and finely dice. Remove mint leave s from stem then chiffon, or thinly slice. Add to strawberries with pepper and squeeze of lime and orange. Mix until well combined.

3   Transfer mixture to serving dish and serve immediately with raw chips. Or refrigerate for 20 minutes and serve chilled.

# Supreme Mango Salsa

Prep Time: 10 minutes

Servings: 4

## INGREDIENTS

2 mangos

1/4 small red onion
1/4 red bell pepper

Small bunch fresh cilantro
1 lime

1/2 fresh jalapeño pepper
1/4 teaspoon Celtic sea salt

## INSTRUCTIONS

1. Slice mangos in half around pit. Remove peel and finely dice flesh. Add to medium mixing bowl.

2. Peel onion and dice. Remove seeds, stem and vein from bell pepper, then finely dice. Finely chop cilantro. Remove seeds and stem from jalapeño, then mince. Add to mango with salt and squeeze of lime. Mix until well combined

3. Transfer mixture to serving dish and serve immediately with raw chips. Or refrigerate for 20 minutes and serve chilled.

# HotApricot Pineapple Salsa

Prep Time: 15 minutes

Servings: 4

INGREDIENTS

1 cup fresh pineapple (diced)

3 fresh apricots

1/2 green bell pepper

1/2 cup cherry tomatoes

2 shallots

2 garlic cloves

1 lime

1 fresh Serrano pepper

Small bunch cilantro leaves

1/2 teaspoon cayenne pepper

1/4 teaspoon Celtic sea salt

INSTRUCTIONS

1. Peel pineapple and finely dice. Cut apricots in half and remove pits, then finely dice. Add to medium mixing bowl.

2. Peel shallots and thinly slice. Peel garlic and mince or thinly slice. Remove seeds, stem and vein from bell pepper, then finely dice. Quarter cherry tomatoes. Add to pineapple and apricot.

3. Finely chop cilantro. Remove seeds and stem from Serrano pepper, then mince. Add to bowl with salt, cayenne and squeeze of lime. Mix until well combined.

4. Transfer mixture to serving dish and serve immediately with raw chips. Or refrigerate for 20 minutes and serve chilled.

# Fresh Zesty Pico de Gallo

Prep Time: 15 minutes*

Servings: 4

INGREDIENTS

4plum tomatoes 1/2

small red onion

Small bunch fresh cilantro

1/2 jalapeño pepper

1/2 lime

1 garlic clove

1/8 teaspoon garlic powder

1/4 teaspoon ground cumin

1/4 teaspoon Celtic sea salt

1/4 teaspoon ground black pepper

INSTRUCTIONS

1. Finely dice tomatoes. Peel and dice onion. Add to medium mixing bowl.

2. Finely chop cilantro. Remove seeds, veins and stem from jalapeño, then mince. Peel and mince garlic. Add to tomatoes with salt, spices and squeeze of lime. Mix until well combined.

3. Transfer mixture to serving dish

4. *Refrigerate 3 hours. Serve room temperature or chilled with raw chips.

# Holy Loaded Guacamole

Prep Time: 5 minutes

Servings: 2

## INGREDIENTS

2 ripe avocados

1 small plum tomato

1/4 small red onion

Medium bunch fresh cilantro

1/2 lime

1/2 teaspoon smoked paprika

1/2 teaspoon ground black pepper

1/2 teaspoon Celtic sea salt

## INSTRUCTIONS

1. Cut avocados in half and remove pits. Scoop flesh into small mixing bowl.

2. Peel onion and dice. Dice tomato. Finely chop cilantro. Add to avocado with salt, spices, and squeeze of lime. Mash with fork until well combined.

3. Transfer mixture to serving dish and serve immediately with raw chips. Or refrigerate for 20 minutes and serve chilled.

# Spicy Stuffed Jalapeños

Prep Time: 15 minutes*

Dehydrating Time: 8 - 24 hours

Servings: 4

## INGREDIENTS

6 fresh jalapeño peppers

1 cup raw sunflower
seeds 1/2 cup water

1/4 cup nutritional yeast

1.lemon

2  teaspoons onion powder
1/2 teaspoon cayenne pepper

5. teaspoon Celtic sea salt
Water

## INSTRUCTIONS

1. *Soak sunflower seeds in enough water to cover for 2 hours. Drain and rinse.

2. Cut jalapeños in half lengthwise and remove stems, seeds and veins. Place peppers on dehydrator tray.

3. Juice lemon. Add to food processor or high-speed blender with soaked sunflower seeds, water, nutritional yeast, salt, pepper and spices. Process until thick, smooth paste forms, about 2 minutes.

4. Fill piping bag with mixture and pipe into jalapeño halves. Or use teaspoon to scoop filling into jalapeño halves.

5. Place stuffed peppers on dehydrator sheets filling-side up. Set dehydrator to 110 degrees F for 8- 24 hours, depending on desired texture.
6. Remove peppers from dehydrator and serve immediately.

Made in the USA
Las Vegas, NV
10 February 2022

43588263R00046